MARK BLOORE

Good Eating with Diabetes

Enjoy Food while Controlling Your Blood Sugar

Copyright © 2025 by mARK bLOORE

All rights reserved. No part of this publication may be reproduced, stored or transmitted in any form or by any means, electronic, mechanical, photocopying, recording, scanning, or otherwise without written permission from the publisher. It is illegal to copy this book, post it to a website, or distribute it by any other means without permission.

First edition

This book was professionally typeset on Reedsy.
Find out more at reedsy.com

Contents

Introduction	1
General Dietary Principles	4
Specific Dietary Advice	10
A Food List	23
In Conclusion	27
Info Sources	29

Introduction

Not medical info or advice

First and foremost, I am not a medical professional of any kind. Please refer your diabetes management to a medical doctor, including dietary changes.

About type 2 diabetes

The point of this book is to show that one can control type 2 diabetes with a good and interesting diet. Too many people believe that a diabetic's diet must be bland. That is not true!

Type 2 diabetes is characterized as a problem of high blood sugar, but really it is a problem of high carbohydrate consumption. Or one could say that it is carbohydrate intolerance, since the body can't handle the amount of carbohydrate being eaten.

Type 2 diabetics can typically keep their blood sugar under control by diet, without needing insulin. Their bodies still make insulin, but they eat more carbs than their bodies can handle. That is usually a result of eating far too much carbohydrate over many years, causing their body to store the excess as fat, until their cells can take no more and stop responding fully to the insulin. That is called insulin resistance, but really it is chronic carbohydrate overload. (Type 1 diabetics must use insulin, since their bodies can not make any at all.)

Based on personal experience

I was diagnosed with type 2 diabetes about 14 years ago. I was lucky and was diagnosed before it had a chance to do much damage. But it is never too late to limit that damage!

After diagnosis I started reading about diabetes, and learned that high blood sugar is the root cause of the many ills diabetes can lead to, everything from swollen feet to losing feet. And the root cause of high blood sugar is diet, in particular sugars and other carbohydrates in food. I also learned that the standard dietary advice for diabetics, along with everyone else, is to get 30% of one's calories from carbs.

For about a year and a half I experimented with various food sources of carbs while avoiding the obviously bad ones, like white bread and sugary beverages. Ancient grains, sprouted grains, spelt, quinoa, nothing let me keep my blood sugar properly controlled. I also tried many heat-and-eat type foods: convenience had been the guiding principle of my diet for many years (which is probably what got me into this state). I finally decided to give up on the 30% rule and on convenience, and eat real food with as little carbs as I could manage. So diabetes is responsible for making me eat a healthy diet!

Working out your own diet

Everyone is different. The details of a diet that works well for me will not be the same for you. To figure out your own personal diet you need to monitor your blood sugar, using a glucometer, or blood glucose meter. You plug a test strip into the meter, prick your finger to get a small drop of blood, and touch it to the strip. A glucose reading appears on the meter a few seconds later. The meter makers get their profit from selling the test strips, so typically you can get the meter for free when you buy a box or two of strips.

When I started I took a glucose reading every morning upon waking, and then one hour and two hours after each meal. That morning reading gave me an idea of how well I was doing overall, and the after-meal readings let me see what particular foods did. These days I still take the morning reading, but usually only bother after meals when trying something new.

Blood glucose levels are reported in two different units, mg/dL (milligrams per deciliter) is usual in the US, and mmol/L (millimoles per litre) everywhere else. Most meters will let you choose the units they show. The commonly recommended maximum values one wants to see are

The lower you can keep those values the better, within limits. The lowest you want to see are

Ideal is to stay in a range of 80-85, or 4.4-4.7 all the time, but this is probably unrealistic.

HbA1c

There is a blood test called hemoglobin A1c, which gives a roughly three-month average of blood sugar, expressed as a percentage of 'glycosylated hemoglobin' in your red blood cells. Blood sugar attaches randomly to proteins in your body (that's the main thing that makes it dangerous), and HbA1c says how much of the protein hemoglobin in your blood has been affected. Red blood cells only last about three months, so this gives an indication of recent history. Usually a value over 7.0% is considered diabetic, and over 6.5% is considered prediabetic. A non-diabetic's value may be 4.0-4.5%, but a diabetic is doing well to keep to about 5.0%.

General Dietary Principles

The defining characteristic of diabetes is an inability to properly handle carbohydrates in one's diet, which leads to high blood sugar. Thus, this book is all about diet and how to use it to control one's blood sugar.

This chapter starts with the official advice, and why one should not follow it.

Official Advice:

The following advice is based on widely accepted guidelines (such as those from the American Diabetes Association). This is what you are likely to hear from a registered dietitian or healthcare professional, as summarized by ChatGPT.

Focus on Balanced, Nutrient-Dense Foods

A key principle of the officially recommended diet for someone with type 2 diabetes is to emphasize whole, minimally processed foods. This includes non-starchy vegetables (like leafy greens, broccoli, and peppers), whole grains (such as oatmeal, brown rice, or whole wheat bread), legumes (beans, lentils), lean protein sources (like fish, poultry, or tofu), and low-fat dairy. These foods generally have a lower glycemic impact than highly processed products, helping to keep blood sugar levels more stable throughout the day. By centering meals around vegetables, whole grains, and lean proteins, individuals can obtain essential vitamins, minerals, and fiber while maintaining better control over their carbohydrate intake.

Carbohydrate Management and Portion Control

Carbohydrates have the most direct impact on blood sugar levels, so managing portion sizes and choosing healthy carb sources are important strategies. Complex carbohydrates with plenty of fiber—such as those found in whole grains, legumes, and certain fruits—tend to be digested more slowly, helping reduce blood sugar spikes. At the same time, limiting or avoiding refined carbohydrates, sugary beverages, and sweets can help keep blood glucose within target ranges. Balancing meals with adequate protein and healthy fats (like avocados, nuts, and olive oil) can further stabilize blood sugar levels and promote satiety. A healthcare provider or registered dietitian may recommend using the "Plate Method," where half the plate is filled with non-starchy vegetables, a quarter with lean protein, and the remaining quarter with whole-grain carbohydrates.

Healthy Fats and Limited Sodium

Choosing monounsaturated and polyunsaturated fats—found in foods such as salmon, tuna, nuts, seeds, and olive oil—can support heart health, which is especially important for individuals with diabetes, as they often face a higher risk of cardiovascular issues. Limiting saturated and trans fats (for example, found in some processed snacks, fried foods, and full-fat dairy) can further help reduce this risk. Monitoring sodium intake is also advisable, as excess salt can contribute to high blood pressure. Aiming for fresh, whole foods and using herbs and spices instead of salt to flavor meals can help manage sodium intake.

Individualization and Monitoring

Although these guidelines provide a strong foundation, dietary needs can vary significantly among people with type 2 diabetes. Factors like activity level, weight goals, medications, and personal preferences all play a role in determining the ideal meal plan. Regularly monitoring blood sugar levels, staying informed about personal nutrition targets, and checking in with healthcare providers help tailor the diet more precisely to an individual's health goals. Regular follow-ups with a registered dietitian can also ensure that any needed adjustments are made over time.

Thoughts:

That is not all bad advice. Nutrient-dense foods are important. Healthy fats are important, but the official guidelines as to what fats are healthy are often wrong, or at best unsettled science; there is still much controversy about saturated fats. Limiting sodium is usually not required if you don't eat salt-laden foods, and limiting it too much is dangerous.

Better Advice: A Low-Carb Diet

Notice that the official advice includes eating a lot of carbs, such as whole grains. All grains are mostly starch, which starts turning into glucose as soon as you chew it. So, avoid grains and everything made from them. The exception is foods high in dietary fibre, with little or no starch or sugar. Fibre is not digestible by humans, but is digestible by your gut microbiome, which in turn provides many benefits.

It is often said that one's body needs carbs, in particular glucose, for energy. That is not true. Most tissues, even the brain, can run on fats, and the ketones derived from them. What little glucose you really need your liver can make from protein, if you don't eat enough carbs (which usually you will – getting to zero carb is very difficult).

Low Carb, High Fat

If you don't eat (much) carbohydrate, you need another source of energy. Fat is your friend. It sounds strange, but eating fat does not make you fat. Eating carbs does. There are many reasons for that, including:

1. It is easy to overeat carbs, and in order to keep excess glucose from causing problems, the cells turn it into fat.
2. If you are eating low carb, your body adapts to burning fat. If you are eating high carb, your body burns the carbs and stores the fat you eat.
3. Eating carbs raises insulin in your blood, and that does two things: it makes your cells take glucose out of the blood, and makes your cells keep the fat they have, rather than burn it for energy.

High insulin, from eating high carb, has other effects, such as encouraging cholesterol deposits in the arteries, i.e. hardening of the arteries.

A low-carb, high-fat (LCHF) diet is a way to help manage your blood sugar. The basic idea behind LCHF is to cut back on foods that are high in carbohydrates—like bread, pasta, and sugary snacks and sodas—since carbs have the biggest impact on your blood sugar levels. Instead, you focus on eating more healthy fats, which have much less of an effect on your glucose readings. By doing this, a lot of people notice more stable energy throughout the day and fewer big spikes or drops in blood sugar. Some even find that they need less of certain diabetes medications (with their doctor's guidance, of course).

Another benefit of LCHF is that it often encourages you to eat more whole, unprocessed foods. When you cut out refined carbs, you tend to load up on veggies, nuts, seeds, and foods like avocados and olives—foods rich in nutrients and fiber. This can make you feel fuller for longer, which might help if you're also trying to manage your weight. Plus, healthy fats—particularly those from sources like meat, fish, nuts, and olive or avocado oil—can be good for heart health, and that's especially important for people with diabetes, who face a higher risk of heart disease.

That said, an LCHF approach isn't the perfect fit for everyone. Some folks love it, while others find it difficult to maintain or discover it just doesn't work well with their lifestyle or medical needs. If you're considering going low-carb, it's super important to keep an eye on your blood sugar levels, because adjusting your carbs can affect the way your medications work. And don't forget that not all fats are created equal. It's best to focus on healthier fats while keeping things like seed oils (e.g. corn, canola) fats to a minimum. Artificial trans fats (aka hydrogenated vegetable oils) are right out, but the small amounts of natural trans fats found in beef and dairy are fine.

If you're thinking about trying a low-carb, high-fat diet, talking to your healthcare team is a smart move. They can help tailor a plan to your specific needs, monitor your progress, and make sure everything's in balance. That way, you can figure out whether LCHF really is the right fit for your diabetes management—and how to do it safely.

Protein

A note about protein: It can be used by the body for energy, but that is not ideal. Your body will use fat and carbs first, but if it runs out of those stores it will break down muscle to get protein. That is because while your body can store limited carb and effectively unlimited fat, it has no protein store besides muscle. So you need to eat protein, preferably at every meal, but overdoing it won't help, and in fact when people have tried very-high-protein diets, say for athletes, they became nauseous and quit. Moderate protein fits with a LCHF diet. Low protein may be unhealthy. As one ages the need for protein increases, to avoid muscle wasting. Of course, exercise is needed too.

Ketogenesis

Ketogenesis is essentially your body's way of making a new fuel source when it doesn't have enough carbohydrates to burn for energy. Picture this: normally, your body uses carbs (like bread, pasta, or fruit) to get the glucose it needs. But if you cut way back on carbs or go for a long stretch without eating—like during an extended fast—your body starts to dip into its fat reserves to keep things running. Your liver breaks down these fats and creates something called "ketone bodies," which can be used as a primary source of energy by your brain and muscles.

There are three main ketones you'll hear about: acetoacetate, beta-hydroxybutyrate (often just called BHB), and acetone. You might notice a distinct "fruity" smell on your breath when your body is producing a lot of acetone—it's one of those telltale signs you're in ketosis. This process can be a big part of diets like keto or LCHF programs, where the goal is to get your body into that fat-burning state.

At the same time, ketogenesis isn't something to take lightly. If you're managing health conditions like diabetes (especially type 1), you've probably been warned about diabetic ketoacidosis (DKA), which is a dangerous state where ketones build up in the blood. That's different from normal ketosis—DKA is a medical emergency. So, if you're thinking about dramatically shifting your carb intake or you're curious about ketosis, it's important to talk with your doctor or dietitian, especially if you have underlying health issues. But many medical professionals and dietitians are unfamiliar with dietary ketosis as opposed to DKA, so some discussion may be needed.

Specific Dietary Advice

High-carb foods

The main sources of carbs are sugars, grains, fruits, starchy vegetables, and processed foods. Except for certain fruits it is best to avoid them all.

There are three main types of carbs: sugars, starches, and fiber. There are many types of simple sugars (monosaccharides), but the ones that are prominent in our diet are glucose, fructose, and galactose. A few sugars are disaccharides: two sugar molecules bonded together. Table sugar, called sucrose, is a glucose bonded to a fructose. Milk sugar, called lactose, is a glucose bonded to a galactose. Starches are many glucose molecules bonded together in a long chain. Fiber is also glucose, and sometimes other molecules, in more complex arrangements.

Not all carbs are the same. Understanding the different types can help you make better food choices, especially if you're managing type 2 diabetes.

Simple Carbohydrates

Simple carbs are like the quick energy snacks of the nutrient world. They're made up of one or two sugar molecules, which means your body can break them down and use them for energy pretty fast. Common simple carbs include glucose, fructose (found in fruits), and lactose (found in dairy). While fruits and dairy products contain simple sugars, they also pack vitamins, minerals, and other beneficial nutrients. On the flip side, simple carbs in sugary drinks, candies, and baked goods often come with little nutritional value and can cause rapid spikes in blood sugar levels, which isn't good for diabetes management, or for health in general.

Fructose

Fructose, fruit sugar, is special, in that it can cause worse trouble than glucose. The amounts found in fruit are fine, but table sugar and high-fructose corn syrup are very common sweeteners, and are half or more fructose. Fructose is only processed in the liver, and if it is overloaded with the stuff, it converts it to fat. Fatty liver disease is the consequence, and it is becoming ever more common as people consume ever more sweet foods and beverages. The good news is that a healthy diet and exercise can take that fat away again.

Complex Carbohydrates

Complex carbs, mostly starches, are made up of longer chains of sugar molecules, which means they take somewhat more time for your body to break down and use. With diabetes that may not make much difference. You'll find complex carbohydrates in foods like whole grains (such as brown rice, quinoa, and whole wheat bread), legumes (beans, lentils, and peas), and starchy vegetables (potatoes, sweet potatoes, and corn). These foods are generally higher in fiber, which is good, but for someone with type 2 diabetes, complex carbs may not really be much better than simple sugars. Best to avoid them.

Dietary Fiber

Fiber plays a crucial role in maintaining a healthy gut microbiome, which in turn has a significant impact on your overall health. Your gut microbiome is a bustling community of trillions of microorganisms living in your digestive system. These microbes help break down the food you eat, produce essential vitamins, and protect against harmful pathogens. Fiber acts as a food for these beneficial bacteria, promoting their growth and activity.

There are two main types of fiber: soluble and insoluble. **Soluble fiber** dissolves in water to form a gel-like substance and is found in foods like oats, beans, and fruits. This type of fiber is especially beneficial for the gut microbiome because it serves as a prebiotic. Prebiotics are non-digestible fibers that feed the good bacteria in your gut, helping them thrive. When these bacteria ferment soluble fiber, they produce short-chain fatty acids (SCFAs) like butyrate, acetate, and propionate. SCFAs are vital for gut health as they help maintain the integrity of the gut lining, reduce inflammation, and provide energy to the cells lining your colon.

Insoluble fiber, found in whole grains, nuts, and vegetables, doesn't dissolve in water but adds bulk to your stool, aiding in regular bowel movements and preventing constipation. While it doesn't directly feed gut bacteria as much as soluble fiber, it still contributes to a healthy digestive system by ensuring that waste moves smoothly through your intestines. A well-functioning digestive system supports overall health by preventing issues like bloating, discomfort, and more serious conditions such as diverticulitis.

Beyond digestion, a healthy gut microbiome influenced by adequate fiber intake has far-reaching effects on your immune system and even your mental health. A balanced microbiome helps regulate immune responses, making your body more efficient at fighting off infections and reducing the risk of autoimmune diseases. Emerging research also suggests a strong connection between gut health and the brain, often referred to as the "gut-brain axis." By supporting a diverse and balanced microbiome, fiber can help improve mood, reduce anxiety, and enhance cognitive functions.

In summary, fiber is essential for nourishing your gut microbiome, which plays a pivotal role in maintaining not just digestive health but also overall well-being. Incorporating a variety of fiber-rich foods into your diet can lead to a healthier gut, a stronger immune system, and better mental health, highlighting the importance of fiber in a balanced and nutritious diet.

Refined Carbohydrates

Refined carbs have been processed to remove the bran and germ, which also strips away fiber, vitamins, and minerals. Examples include white bread, white rice, and many breakfast cereals. Because they lack fiber, refined carbs can cause quicker spikes in blood sugar compared to their whole counterparts. For those managing type 2 diabetes, it's usually better to avoid refined carbohydrates even more than complex carbs.

Natural vs. Added Sugars

Natural sugars are found naturally in foods like fruits, vegetables, and dairy products. Added sugars, on the other hand, are those that manufacturers add to foods and beverages during processing or preparation, such as in sodas, sweets, and many packaged snacks. The may also be present in things which don't taste sweet, but which might taste bad without them. Your body does not care whether sugars were added or original, the effect on your blood sugar only depends on the total amount of sugar.

Understanding the different types of carbohydrates and how they affect your body can empower you to make healthier choices and better manage your blood sugar levels. It's always a good idea to talk with a healthcare provider or a registered dietitian to create a carb plan that works best for your individual needs.

Low-carb foods

Low-carb foods include meat, seafood, eggs, cheese, leafy greens, nuts, certain fruits, and many others. Keep a watch out for good eating that is low carb. There are many choices.

Anything animal-based will have no carbs, or at most a tiny amount. Usually it will have complete protein, meaning all the essential amino acids are present.

Root vegetables, such as potatoes, are mostly starch, i.e. carbs. The same is true of grains, like corn, wheat, oats, and rice. Starch starts turning into glucose as soon as you chew it.

Most fruits contain a lot of sugar. Important exceptions are avocados, which have good fats and fibre, and berries, which contain a little sugar along with substances which make your tongue think there is a lot of sugar. Berries have a lot of valuable nutrients in them.

Fat types:

Fats and oils, also called fatty acids, are major sources of energy in your body, and also components of every cell, especially in the brain. They are vital, but not all are good.

Saturated Fatty Acids

Think of saturated fats (SFAs) as the "solid" fats you find in things like butter, cheese, and red meat. They're also in some plant-based oils like coconut and palm oil. These fats are pretty stable, which is why they stay solid at room temperature. For decades saturated fats were villainized as the cause of heart disease. Research over many recent years has shown them to be necessary rather than dangerous, but the old fear of fat lingers.

Unsaturated Fatty Acids

Unsaturated fats are the "liquid" fats, usually found in oils like olive, canola, and sunflower. They're split into two main groups: monounsaturated and polyunsaturated fats.

- **Monounsaturated Fats (MUFAs):** These are the good guys you find in olive oil, avocados, and nuts like almonds and cashews. MUFAs can help lower your "bad" LDL cholesterol while keeping the good HDL cholesterol up. (But, like SFA, LDL cholesterol is starting to look like it's not so bad, especially for people on a LCHF diet.) Plus, they make your meals more satisfying, which can help with weight management.
- **Polyunsaturated Fats (PUFAs):** These include omega-3 and omega-6 fatty acids, which are essential for your body because you can't make them yourself. Omega-3s, especially EPA and DHA, are awesome for your heart and brain and are found in fatty fish like salmon, as well as in grass-fed beef (but not grain-fed. Grass has omega-3s, but grain has only omega-6s, and all that gets passed into the meat and milk.) Various plant sources, such as flaxseeds and walnuts, contain short-chain omega-3s (ALA), which your body

needs some of, but your body can only convert a very small amount of ALA into EPA and DHA, so you need those in your diet. Omega-6s are in vegetable oils and nuts, but it's important to keep a good balance between omega-3 and omega-6 to avoid inflammation.
- **Seed Oils:** Seed or vegetable oils, such as corn, canola, sunflower, grapeseed, and others, are heavily processed with heat and solvents. As a result they are oxidized and unhealthy. They produce reactive oxygen species in your body, which are the very thing you are trying to reduce by eating antioxidants! Avoid them, unless you can find 'virgin cold-pressed' types.

Trans Fatty Acids

Trans fats are the villains in the fatty acid world. They're artificially created through a process called hydrogenation, which turns liquid oils into solid fats. You used to find them in processed foods like margarine, snack foods, and baked goods. Trans fats are bad news because they raise your bad LDL cholesterol and lower your good HDL cholesterol, significantly increasing the risk of heart disease and other health issues. They may also replace natural fats in places like cell membranes, where they cause problems. It's best to avoid trans fats entirely by checking food labels and steering clear of anything with partially hydrogenated oils. Note that beef and dairy contain small amounts of natural trans fats, which do not appear to be a problem. If a nutrition label mentions trans fats, look at the ingredients list to see where they came from.

Other Types of Fatty Acids

- **Essential Fatty Acids:** These include both omega-3 and omega-6 fats. Since your body can't produce them, you need to get them from your diet. They're crucial for brain function, cell growth, and

regulating inflammation.
- **Short-Chain and Medium-Chain Fatty Acids:** Found in foods like dairy products and coconut oil, these fats are easier for your body to digest and can be quickly used for energy.

Wrapping It Up

Understanding the different types of fatty acids can really help you make better food choices. Focusing on healthy fats, especially those rich in omega-3s, while keeping other polyunsaturated fats in check and avoiding trans fats, can boost your heart health and overall well-being. As always, chatting with a healthcare professional or a registered dietitian can help you figure out the best fat intake for your personal health goals. But be aware that old ideas about the evils of saturated fats persist, even among professionals.

Fat sources:

Animal

Animal fatty acids are mostly saturated (SFA), which is fine, despite the "common wisdom". They also include omega fatty acids, and there's something to watch out for: animals don't make omega fatty acids, they only get it from their food. Grasses have both omega-3 and omega-6, but grains have only omega-6. So fat from grass-fed animals will have a good mix of omegas, but fat from grain-fed or grain-finished animals will have too much omega-6s for good health.

Seafood, especially fatty fish like salmon, herring, sardines, and others, is a good source of omega-3s, and of protein also.

Plant

Plant fatty acids are mostly mono- and poly-unstaturated. Mono unsaturated (MUFA) are generally good for your health. Poly unsaturated (PUFA) are often bad. An exception is the omega fatty acids, which you must eat. But PUFA is easily oxidized, i.e. made rancid, which makes them unhealthy. Industrial production of such oils, like corn, canola, and sunflower, uses high temperature and solvents to extract as much as possible from the source. That leaves them oxidized when you buy them. If you can find oils marked 'cold pressed' and 'virgin', they should be in a better state. But keep them in a cool, dark place. The same goes for generally healthy oils, like olive and avocado.

Coconut oil has a lot of saturated fatty acids, but they are smaller than the animal types, which means that even if animal fats are bad, coconut oil may not be. Those short-chain fatty acids are good food for your gut microbiome.

Fermented foods

Fermented foods are those that have gone through a natural process where bacteria, yeast, or other microorganisms break down the sugars and starches. Think yogurt, kimchi, sauerkraut, kefir, kombucha, and even some types of pickles. This process not only preserves the food but also boosts its nutritional profile.

Probiotics Power

One of the biggest benefits of fermented foods is that they're packed with probiotics—the good bacteria that live in your gut. These friendly microbes help keep your digestive system running smoothly, improve nutrient absorption, create nutrients such as some vitamins, and even support your immune system. A healthy gut microbiome is linked to better digestion, reduced inflammation, and can even impact your mood and energy levels.

Enhanced Nutrient Content

Fermentation can increase the availability of certain vitamins and minerals in foods. For example, it can boost levels of B vitamins, vitamin K, and some antioxidants. This means your body can absorb and use these nutrients more effectively compared to their non-fermented counterparts.

Better Digestion

If you've ever felt bloated or had trouble digesting certain foods, fermented options might be a game-changer. The probiotics and the breakdown of food during fermentation make these foods easier to digest. This can be especially helpful for people with lactose intolerance, as fermentation reduces the lactose content in dairy products like yogurt and kefir.

Natural Preservation and Flavor Boost

Fermentation naturally preserves foods without the need for artificial additives. Plus, it adds unique, tangy flavors that can make your meals more interesting and delicious. Whether it's the zing of sauerkraut on your sausage or the creamy tang of yogurt in your smoothie, fermented foods can elevate your dishes both taste-wise and health-wise.

Potential Immune Support

A healthy gut is closely linked to a strong immune system. By supporting your gut health with fermented foods, you're also giving your immune system a boost. Some studies suggest that regular consumption of probiotics can help reduce the frequency and duration of certain infections.

In a Nutshell

Incorporating fermented foods into your diet is a tasty and effective way to enhance your nutrition. They provide beneficial probiotics for gut health, improve digestion, increase nutrient availability, and add delicious flavors to your meals. Whether you're adding some kimchi to your meal or enjoying a glass of kombucha, fermented foods can be a fantastic addition to a balanced and healthy diet.

Processed foods

Processed foods are pretty much anything that isn't straight from the farm or garden. They are ubiquitous in the Standard American Diet (appropriately known as SAD). Fermented foods are processed, but are usually quite healthy, avoiding the problems described here.

Loaded with Unhealthy Ingredients

Processed foods often come packed with added sugars, unhealthy fats, and high levels of sodium. Think about your favorite chips, sugary cereals, or fast food meals—they're tasty but can contribute to weight gain, high blood pressure, and increased cholesterol levels when eaten regularly. These ingredients are added to enhance flavor and shelf life but aren't great for your body in the long run.

Low in Nutrients

While processed foods might be convenient, they're usually stripped of essential nutrients like fiber, vitamins, and minerals. Instead of getting the nutrients your body needs, you're getting empty calories that don't do much to keep you healthy. This can lead to deficiencies and make it harder to maintain a balanced diet.

Additives and Preservatives

To keep processed foods fresh and appealing, manufacturers add various preservatives, artificial colors, and flavors. Some of these additives have been linked to health issues like allergies, digestive problems, and even behavioral changes in some people. Plus, relying on these additives can make it harder for your body to process natural foods properly.

Impact on Gut Health

Processed foods often lack the fiber that's essential for a healthy gut microbiome. Without enough fiber, your digestion can suffer, leading to issues like constipation and a less diverse population of beneficial gut bacteria. A healthy gut is crucial for everything from digestion to immune function and even your mood.

Increased Risk of Chronic Diseases

Regularly consuming processed foods has been linked to a higher risk of developing chronic diseases such as type 2 diabetes, heart disease, and certain cancers. The combination of unhealthy fats, sugars, and additives can create an environment in your body that promotes inflammation and other harmful processes.

Addictive Qualities

Processed foods are often engineered to be hyper-palatable, meaning they're designed to taste really good and keep you coming back for more. This can lead to overeating and make it harder to maintain a healthy weight. The high levels of sugar, fat, and salt can trigger reward centers in your brain, similar to how addictive substances work.

In a Nutshell

While processed foods are convenient and tasty, they come with several health risks if consumed too often. For diabetics they are a health risk in any amount, due to the carb content. They're typically high in unhealthy ingredients, low in essential nutrients, and can negatively impact your gut health and overall well-being. Opting for whole, minimally processed foods whenever possible is a great way to support your health and feel your best.

A Food List

Here are a few healthy low-carb, and hence diabetic-friendly, foods, in no particular order. There are many more for you to find!

VEGETABLES

- turnip greens
- coriander (cilantro)
- rosemary
- spinach
- parsley
- chives
- peppers / capsicum
- artichokes
- collards
- mushrooms
- Swiss chard
- mustard greens
- broccoli
- Brussels sprouts
- kale
- red or green bell peppers

FATS AND OILS

- grass-fed butter
- coconut oil
- olive oil
- fish oil
- flaxseed oil
- algae oil

Algae oil is a good vegan source of omega-3 fatty acids.

FRUITS

- avocados
- olives
- blueberries
- blackberries
- strawberries
- raspberries

Berries may taste sweet, but they don't really have a lot of sugar. Get wild berries if you can.

EGGS & DAIRY

- whole eggs
- goat cheese
- Parmigiano Reggiano cheese
- cheddar cheese
- cream
- Camembert cheese

- feta cheese
- cream cheese
- blue cheese
- Colby cheese
- Swiss cheese
- Edam cheese
- brie cheese
- Gouda cheese
- mozzarella cheese
- ricotta cheese
- cottage cheese

Free-range eggs are much more nutritious than the usual factory-farmed ones. The chickens are better off, too.

NUTS & SEEDS

- brazil nuts
- sunflower seeds
- pecans
- pumpkin seeds
- almonds
- macadamia nuts
- pine nuts
- coconut milk
- coconut meat
- coconut butter
- pistachio nuts
- cashews

Brazil nuts are good, but go easy. One can overdose on selenium with more than about two nuts per day.

ANIMAL PRODUCTS

- organ meats (liver, kidney, heart, etc)
- chorizo
- bratwurst
- herring
- chicken
- frankfurter
- mackerel
- duck
- grass-fed beef
- turkey
- anchovy
- lamb
- salmon
- bison
- sardines
- pork

There's a lot more nutrition in organ meats than the muscle meat of the animal. And with regular meat, don't cut off the fat or go for low-fat options.

In Conclusion

Eat well and avoid carbs

You may have to avoid your favorite bread, pasta, and cake, but you can eat well and stay healthy despite having type 2 diabetes.

Do research

There is a great deal of information and advice to be found online. (And in books, for that matter.) Just be careful that your sources are educated and not only looking to sell you stuff.

Find others online

Facebook groups, YouTube channels, and many other gathering places will include ones made by and for diabetics.

Leave a book review!

If you found this little book helpful, please leave a positive review on Amazon.

Info Sources

There are many sources of diabetes info, online and off. These are just a few.

- Examine®: Looks at research into many dietary supplements. http://examine.com
- Physionic: A PhD candidate in molecular medicine examines health-related research papers. http://physionic.mn.co
- GlucoseRevolution: Talks about many diabetes topics https://www.youtube.com/@GlucoseRevolution
- Dr. Boz is an MD who talks about diabetes and other health matters https://www.youtube.com/@DoctorBoz
- Optimising Nutrition: Lots of nutrition info. In particular about type 2 diabetes: https://optimisingnutrition.wordpress.com/2015/03/22/ketosis-the-cure-for-diabetes/
- Gary Taubes, author of a number of books, including *Good Calories, Bad Calories*.
- *Blood Sugar 101*, by Jenny Ruhl. An introduction to dealing with diabetes.
- Dr. Richard K. Bernstein, MD, author of books on handling diabetes, including *Dr. Bernsein's Diabetes Solution*. The author has been type 1 diabetic for a long time.

www.ingramcontent.com/pod-product-compliance
Lightning Source LLC
LaVergne TN
LVHW011004060225
803045LV00003B/287